Managing Diabetes: Understanding and Controlling Type 1, Type 2, and Gestational Diabetes, Practical Strategies for Blood Sugar Management and Lifestyle Adaptation

The Comprehensive Health Series

Dr Paul Sterling

Published by NovaLife Medical Research Center, 2023.

While every precaution has been taken in the preparation of this book, the publisher assumes no responsibility for errors or omissions, or for damages resulting from the use of the information contained herein.

MANAGING DIABETES: UNDERSTANDING AND CONTROLLING TYPE 1, TYPE 2, AND GESTATIONAL DIABETES, PRACTICAL STRATEGIES FOR BLOOD SUGAR MANAGEMENT AND LIFESTYLE ADAPTATION

First edition. November 12, 2023.

ISBN: 979-8215800249

Written by Dr Paul Sterling.

Also by Dr Paul Sterling

The Comprehensive Health Series

Mastering Gastritis: Comprehensive Guide to Understanding and Treating Acute, Chronic, and Erosive Gastritis, plus Stomach Inflammation Management

Managing Diabetes: Understanding and Controlling Type 1, Type 2, and Gestational Diabetes, Practical Strategies for Blood Sugar Management and Lifestyle Adaptation

Table of Contents

Preface

It is an honor to welcome you to *"Managing Diabetes: Understanding and Controlling Type 1, Type 2, and Gestational Diabetes, Practical Strategies for Blood Sugar Management and Lifestyle Adaptation", an informative* resource designed to provide accurate and practical guidance to those who face the daily challenge of living with diabetes. In these pages, you will find a compendium of sound medical knowledge, effective management strategies, and practical advice to help you take control of your health and live a full, active life.

Diabetes may seem overwhelming at first, but we are here to tell you that you are not alone on this journey. This book has been created with care and dedication by medical experts and health professionals, with the aim of providing you with reliable and comprehensive guidance. Every word you'll find here has been carefully selected to offer you accurate, clear information, free of complicated medical jargon, and filled with empathy for the unique experiences each of you face.

Our intention is not only to inform, but also to empower you. Diabetes should not limit your dreams, aspirations or quality of life. Rather than viewing this condition as a barrier, we encourage you to view it as a surmountable challenge. With the right knowledge and the right tools, they can face each day with confidence and determination.

This book will provide them with a detailed understanding of the different types of diabetes, from type 1 to type 2 and gestational diabetes. They will learn about the underlying causes, diagnostic methods, and available treatment options. Additionally, we'll explore the practical aspects of daily management, from meal planning and glucose monitoring to the importance of exercise and stress management.

We will not stop at the purely medical. We will also address the emotional aspects of living with diabetes. We know that mental health is just as important as physical health, and we will provide you with strategies to stay positive and motivated, even in the most challenging times.

Each page of this book has been created with you, your needs and concerns in mind. We encourage you to use it as a practical tool, referring to it whenever you need it and applying the knowledge acquired in your daily life. Remember that even though you face a chronic condition, you have the power to control it and live a full life.

So, dear readers, we welcome you to this journey towards a healthy and controlled life. With every page you read, we hope you find inspiration, guidance, and, above all, hope. Together, we will face diabetes and build a future full of well-being and possibilities.

With warm regards and best wishes,

Dr. Paul Sterling

Introduction

Diabetes, a chronic disease characterized by high blood glucose levels, presents significant challenges for those who suffer from it. This book, "Manage Your Diabetes," focuses on providing accurate and clear medical information as well as practical strategies to help you effectively manage this condition and live a healthy, fulfilling life.

In the pages that follow, you'll find a detailed exploration of the different types of diabetes, including type 1, type 2, and gestational diabetes. We'll break down the underlying causes of each type and the differences in treatment approaches. Additionally, we will delve into potential complications and how to prevent or manage them effectively.

The book will also address fundamental aspects of daily diabetes management, from meal planning and glucose monitoring to the importance of regular exercise and stress management. We will provide you with specific medical advice on how to adapt your lifestyle and habits to maintain stable blood glucose levels.

In the chapters dedicated to employment and education, we will guide you about your rights and reasonable accommodations that can be made in the work and educational environment. It is essential that you understand your rights and how to advocate for them to ensure a supportive environment at work and in the classroom.

Additionally, we will delve into the emotional aspect of living with diabetes. This condition can often lead to stress, anxiety and depression. We will address these concerns and provide you with strategies to stay positive and stay motivated even in the most challenging times.

This book has been created with a rigorous medical approach and clear words to provide you with accurate and reliable information. We reject metaphors and analogies in favor of direct and understandable communication. Each advice and recommendation is based on solid scientific evidence and supported by expert medical professionals in the field of diabetes.

As you read these pages, we encourage you to take a proactive approach to your health. Diabetes shouldn't stop you from living a full and meaningful life. With the right knowledge and the determination to apply it, you can take control of your health and effectively manage this chronic condition.

This book is a valuable tool that will equip you with the knowledge necessary to navigate the challenge of diabetes with confidence and determination. We're here to provide you with the tools and information you need to live a healthy, active life, even as you face diabetes. Together, we will address this condition with understanding and determination, moving towards a healthier and more controlled future.

1.1 Definition and Types of Diabetes:

Diabetes is a chronic condition that affects the way the body uses glucose, a type of sugar that is our main source of energy. To understand it better, it is essential to know the different types of diabetes and how they develop.

- **Type 1 Diabetes:** Type 1 diabetes is a form of autoimmune diabetes. In this condition, the body's immune system attacks and destroys the beta cells in the pancreas, which are responsible for producing insulin. Insulin is crucial for allowing glucose to enter cells and provide energy. Without enough insulin, blood glucose levels rise, which can lead to serious health problems. People with type 1 diabetes need daily insulin injections to control their glucose levels.
- **Type 2 Diabetes:** Type 2 diabetes is the most common form of diabetes and usually develops in adulthood, although it can also affect children and adolescents. In type 2 diabetes, the body does not produce enough insulin or the cells do not respond properly to the insulin that is produced. This is known as insulin resistance. Type 2 diabetes is often linked to obesity and a sedentary lifestyle. Although diet and exercise can help control this form of diabetes, sometimes oral medications or insulin injections are needed.

- **Gestational Diabetes:** Gestational diabetes occurs during pregnancy when the body cannot produce enough extra insulin to meet the body's needs. This can cause high blood glucose levels. Gestational diabetes can increase the risk for both mother and baby, but with proper management, it usually resolves after delivery.
- **Monogenic Diabetes and Other Types: In addition to the main types mentioned, there are less common forms of diabetes, such as** monogenic diabetes , which is caused by a single genetic mutation. There is also secondary diabetes, which develops as a result of other medical conditions, such as diseases of the pancreas or the use of certain medications.

Understanding these types of diabetes is essential for effective management of the disease. Each type requires specific approaches to treatment, monitoring, and lifestyle. In the following pages, we will explore in detail strategies for managing each type, providing essential knowledge and empowering readers to live a full, healthy life despite this chronic condition.

1.2 Causes and Risk Factors of Diabetes

Diabetes is a complex condition, and its development can be influenced by various causes and risk factors. Understanding these elements essentially provides us with the necessary tools for the prevention and proper management of this chronic disease.

Causes:

- **Genetics:** Genetic predisposition plays a crucial role in the development of diabetes. If you have close family members with diabetes, you are more likely to be at risk of developing it as well.
- **Autoimmunity:** In type 1 diabetes, the immune system mistakenly attacks the insulin-producing cells in the pancreas. Although it is not fully understood why this occurs, genetic and environmental factors are thought to play a role.

- **Insulin Resistance:** In type 2 diabetes, the body can produce insulin, but the cells do not respond properly to this hormone. This insulin resistance can be caused by genetic and lifestyle factors, such as obesity and lack of physical activity.

Risk factor's:

- **Obesity:** Obesity, especially excess abdominal fat, is one of the main risk factors for type 2 diabetes. Abdominal fat can cause insulin resistance, leading to elevated blood glucose levels.
- **Physical Inactivity:** Lack of regular physical activity can contribute to the development of type 2 diabetes. Regular exercise not only helps with weight control, but also improves insulin sensitivity.
- **Unbalanced Diet:** Eating foods high in calories, saturated fats and processed sugars increases the risk of diabetes. A diet rich in fruits, vegetables, whole grains, and lean proteins is essential for preventing type 2 diabetes.
- **Family History:** As mentioned above, having family members with diabetes significantly increases the risk. Genetics can play an important role in predisposition to the disease.
- **Age and Ethnicity:** The risk of type 2 diabetes increases with age, especially after age 45. Additionally, certain ethnic groups, such as African Americans, Hispanics, Native Americans, and Asian Americans, are at higher risk.
- **High Blood Pressure and Elevated Cholesterol:** Hypertension and elevated levels of LDL ("bad") cholesterol are linked to an increased risk of developing type 2 diabetes.

It is vital to take these risk factors into account and work on their prevention. Adopting a healthy lifestyle that includes a balanced diet, regular physical activity and weight management can make a big difference in reducing the risk of diabetes. Additionally, awareness of family history and regular medical checkups can help in early detection and effective management of this chronic disease.

CHAPTER 1 : Understanding the types of diabetes

2.1 Type 1 Diabetes: Causes, Symptoms and Treatment:

Type 1 diabetes is a chronic medical condition that affects people of all ages, although it is often diagnosed in childhood or adolescence. Unlike type 2 diabetes, in which the body develops insulin resistance or does not produce enough insulin to meet the body's needs, type 1 diabetes is characterized by an autoimmune response that attacks and destroys beta cells in the pancreas. . These cells are responsible for producing insulin, a hormone essential to allowing cells to absorb and use glucose from the blood as an energy source.

Causes:

The exact cause of type 1 diabetes is not fully understood, but a combination of genetic and environmental factors are thought to play a role in its development. Certain genes are known to increase susceptibility to type 1 diabetes, but not all people with these genes develop the disease. Furthermore, it has been observed that viral infections and environmental factors can trigger the autoimmune response that leads to the destruction of beta cells.

Symptoms:

The symptoms of type 1 diabetes can come on suddenly and be intense. Some of the most common symptoms include:

- **Increased Thirst and Urination:** Due to high blood glucose levels, the body tries to eliminate excess sugar through urine, which can lead to unusually intense thirst and frequent urination, especially at night. .
- **Excessive Hunger:** Despite eating regularly, people with type 1 diabetes may experience constant hunger. This is because the body's cells cannot properly absorb glucose, leading to a persistent feeling of hunger.

- **Unintentional Weight Loss: Unexplained** weight loss is a classic symptom of type 1 diabetes. The body turns to breaking down fat and muscle for energy, leading to weight loss even when you eat the most. enough.
- **Fatigue and Weakness:** The lack of glucose reaching the cells to be used for energy can cause constant fatigue and muscle weakness, even after adequate rest.
- **Changes in Mood:** Imbalances in glucose levels can affect mood, causing irritability, sudden emotional changes and difficulty concentrating.
- **Blurred Vision:** High blood glucose levels can affect the way the eye focuses, leading to blurred vision.
- **Common Infections:** Type 1 diabetes can weaken the immune system, making people more prone to infections, especially of the skin, gums, and urinary tract.
- Treatment:
- The main treatment for type 1 diabetes involves daily administration of insulin. People with this form of diabetes must inject insulin several times a day or use an insulin pump that releases controlled doses throughout the day. The goal is to keep blood glucose levels within a normal range to prevent long-term complications.

In addition to insulin, managing type 1 diabetes involves constant monitoring of blood glucose levels, a balanced diet, and regular participation in physical activities. Continuing education about the disease and emotional support are essential to helping people with type 1 diabetes lead full and active lives, despite the challenges this chronic condition presents. With the right treatment and support, people with type 1 diabetes can lead healthy, productive lives.

2.2 Type 2 Diabetes: Risk Factors and Prevention:

Type 2 diabetes is a chronic condition that affects how the body uses insulin or, in some cases, does not produce enough insulin to keep blood glucose levels within a normal range. Unlike type 1 diabetes, which generally develops in childhood or adolescence, type 2 diabetes is usually diagnosed in adults, although it is becoming more common in younger people due to lifestyle changes.

Risk factor's:

Several factors increase the risk of developing type 2 diabetes. One of the most significant risk factors is obesity, especially when excess fat accumulates around the abdomen. Fat cells, especially those found in the abdominal area, release chemicals that can cause insulin resistance, making it difficult for the cells to absorb glucose.

Lack of physical activity is another important risk factor. Regular exercise not only helps control weight, but also improves insulin sensitivity, allowing cells to use glucose more efficiently.

An unbalanced diet, high in calories, saturated fats and processed sugars, also contributes to the risk of type 2 diabetes. Excessive consumption of processed foods and sugary drinks can increase blood glucose levels and lead to the development of the disease.

A family history of type 2 diabetes also increases the likelihood of developing the disease. If you have parents or siblings with type 2 diabetes, it is important to pay attention to risk factors and adopt a healthy lifestyle to reduce your chances of developing the disease.

Prevention:

The good news is that type 2 diabetes in many cases can be prevented or delayed with lifestyle changes. Weight loss, even a modest loss, and increased physical activity can make a big difference. Even losing 5-10% of body weight can significantly reduce the risk of developing type 2 diabetes.

Adopting a balanced and nutritious diet is key to prevention. Instead of processed and sugary foods, high-fiber foods such as fruits, vegetables, whole grains, and lean proteins should be included in your diet. Avoiding excess calories and saturated fat is also essential for maintaining a healthy weight and reducing the risk of diabetes.

Regular physical activity is essential to prevent type 2 diabetes. At least 150 minutes of moderate aerobic exercise or 75 minutes of vigorous exercise per week is recommended, along with muscle-strengthening activities at least twice a week.

In addition to these lifestyle changes, it is essential to have regular medical checkups to monitor blood glucose levels and other risk factors. Early detection and proper management of risk factors can make a difference in preventing type 2 diabetes and promoting a healthy, active life.

2.3 Gestational Diabetes: Management During Pregnancy:

Gestational diabetes is a type of diabetes that develops during pregnancy. It affects some women who did not have diabetes before pregnancy. Although gestational diabetes usually goes away after childbirth, it can have significant effects on the health of the mother and baby. Proper management of gestational diabetes during pregnancy is essential to ensure a positive outcome for both mother and baby.

Diagnosis and Control:

Diagnosis of gestational diabetes is usually made between weeks 24 and 28 of pregnancy by testing fasting glucose and monitoring blood glucose after drinking a glucose solution. If gestational diabetes is diagnosed, it is crucial to begin proper control of glucose levels.

Control is achieved through changes in diet and exercise, and in some cases, oral medications or insulin may be required. The goal is to maintain blood glucose levels within a normal range to avoid complications for mother and baby.

Glucose Monitoring:

During pregnancy, constant monitoring of blood glucose levels is required to ensure that they are under control. This is accomplished by self-testing your glucose at home with a glucose meter. Daily glucose records help doctors adjust treatment as needed.

Diet and Nutrition:

A fundamental part of managing gestational diabetes is maintaining a balanced diet. Pregnant women with gestational diabetes should follow a diet that controls the amount and type of carbohydrates, and that includes lean proteins, healthy fats, and a variety of fruits and vegetables.

Portion control and tracking carbohydrate intake are key. High-fiber foods, such as whole grains, legumes, and vegetables, are excellent choices for keeping blood glucose levels stable.

Physical exercise:

Regular exercise is beneficial for both pregnant women and the management of gestational diabetes. Moderate physical activity, such as walking or swimming, is recommended for at least 30 minutes a day. Exercise helps maintain a healthy weight and improves insulin sensitivity.

Medications and Insulin:

In some cases, control of gestational diabetes is not achieved through diet and exercise alone, and oral medications or insulin may be required to keep blood glucose levels under control. These medications are used under the supervision of a doctor and healthcare team.

Prenatal Monitoring:

During pregnancy, women with gestational diabetes require closer prenatal monitoring. This includes regular visits to the doctor and possibly an endocrinologist. Ultrasounds are also performed to monitor the baby's growth and health.

Risks and Complications:

If gestational diabetes is not properly controlled, it can lead to complications for the mother and baby. Some of the complications include:

- **Excessive fetal growth:** Uncontrolled gestational diabetes can lead to excessive growth of the baby, which may require a cesarean delivery.

- **Neonatal hypoglycemia:** Babies born to mothers with poorly controlled gestational diabetes may experience low blood glucose levels after birth.
- **High blood pressure and preeclampsia** : Pregnant women with gestational diabetes are at increased risk of developing high blood pressure and preeclampsia .
- **Premature birth:** Gestational diabetes can increase the risk of preterm birth.

Proper management of gestational diabetes during pregnancy is essential to prevent complications and ensure a positive outcome for mother and baby. Following medical recommendations and self-care are essential for a healthy and successful pregnancy

CHAPTER 3: Diagnosis and monitoring

3.1 Diagnostic methods

Early and accurate diagnosis of diabetes is essential for effective management and prevention of long-term complications. Over the years, several methods have been developed to diagnose diabetes and assess blood glucose levels. These methods are essential to determine the type of diabetes and establish an appropriate treatment plan.

- Fasting Glucose Tests:

One of the most common tests to diagnose diabetes is the fasting glucose test. This test is performed after a period of overnight fasting and measures blood glucose levels at that time. If results show fasting glucose levels equal to or greater than 126 mg/ dL on two separate tests, the diagnosis of diabetes is confirmed.

- Hemoglobin A1c Test:

The hemoglobin A1c test is another important tool for diagnosing diabetes. This test provides a measure of blood sugar control over the past two to three months by assessing the percentage of hemoglobin that has been affected by blood sugar. An A1c result of 6.5% or higher confirms the diagnosis of diabetes.

- Oral Glucose Tolerance Test:

The oral glucose tolerance test involves drinking a glucose solution and measuring blood glucose levels two hours later. This test is used to evaluate how the body processes glucose. A result equal to or greater than 200 mg/ dL two hours after drinking the solution confirms the diagnosis of diabetes.

- Postprandial Glucose Tests :

Postprandial glucose tests are done two hours after eating a meal. Postprandial glucose levels help evaluate how the body handles sugar after meals. If the results show glucose levels equal to or greater than 200 mg/ dL , it may indicate diabetes.

- Continuous Glucose Monitoring:

Continuous glucose monitoring (CGM) is a newer technology that involves using a sensor under the skin to measure glucose levels in real time throughout the day. The data collected provides detailed information about how food, exercise, and other factors affect blood sugar levels. Although not used for initial diagnosis, CGM is vital for the long-term management of diabetes.

Early and accurate diagnosis of diabetes is essential for effective management and to prevent long-term complications. Fasting glucose testing, hemoglobin A1c, oral glucose tolerance, and postprandial glucose testing are key tools in diagnosing diabetes and determining the specific type of the disease. Additionally, continuous glucose monitoring provides valuable information for daily disease management. Timely diagnosis and proper care allow people with diabetes to lead active, healthy lives while controlling their blood glucose levels effectively.

3.2 Importance of regular monitoring

Regular monitoring of blood glucose levels is an essential practice for people living with diabetes. It is often said that control is power, and in the case of diabetes, this is especially true. Regular monitoring not only provides vital information about how the body responds to food, exercise and medication, but also plays a crucial role in preventing long-term complications.

- Custom Control:

Each person is unique, and the way diabetes affects your body can vary widely. Regular monitoring allows for a personalized understanding of how food, physical activity, and other factors affect blood glucose levels. By regularly recording blood sugar levels and observed patterns, people with diabetes and their doctors can adjust treatment and lifestyle specifically to meet their individual needs. This not only improves glycemic control, but also helps prevent diabetes-related complications.

- Prevention of Complications:

One of the biggest risks associated with poorly controlled diabetes is long-term complications. These can include heart disease, kidney damage, eye problems, neuropathy, and foot ulcers. Without proper control of blood glucose levels, these problems can arise and significantly affect quality of life. However, regular monitoring can detect any unusual increases in glucose levels and take steps to prevent complications before they become serious problems.

- Empowerment and Awareness:

Regular monitoring not only provides data for healthcare professionals, but also empowers people with diabetes by giving them greater control over their health. By being aware of their blood glucose levels and understanding how food, exercise, and other factors affect these levels, people with diabetes can make informed decisions about their lifestyle and treatment. This awareness can lead to better decision-making regarding diet, medication, and physical activity, which in turn improves quality of life and overall well-being.

- Promotion of Self-Care:

Regular monitoring promotes a culture of self-care in people with diabetes. By taking an active role in managing their condition, people with diabetes can learn to recognize the warning signs of abnormal glucose levels and take quick steps to correct them. This may include dietary adjustments, medication dosages, or additional physical activity. Empowering self-care not only benefits physical health, but can also have a positive impact on mental health by reducing stress and anxiety related to illness.

Regular monitoring of blood glucose levels is essential for effective diabetes management. It provides personalized information, prevents long-term complications, empowers people with diabetes, promotes a culture of self-care and improves overall quality of life. By incorporating regular monitoring as a routine practice, people with diabetes can live full, healthy lives while effectively managing their condition.

CHAPTER 4: Lifestyle Management
4.1 Meal planning and balanced diet

Meal planning and a balanced diet are crucial components in effective diabetes management. When living with this chronic condition, what you eat and how meals are planned can make a big difference in blood glucose levels, weight management, and ultimately quality of life. Through a well-balanced diet and careful planning, people with diabetes can control their blood sugar levels, prevent complications, and enjoy a healthy, active life.

- Importance of Meal Planning:

Careful meal planning is essential for people with diabetes. Instead of focusing solely on calorie restriction, the focus is on choosing foods that help keep blood glucose levels within a healthy range. This involves careful consideration of the carbohydrates, fats, proteins, fiber and micronutrients in each meal.

- Carbohydrate Control:

Carbohydrates have a direct impact on blood glucose levels. Therefore, it is essential to control the amount and type of carbohydrates consumed. Opting for complex, low-glycemic carbohydrates, such as whole grains, legumes, and vegetables, helps keep blood glucose stable. Additionally, it is important to distribute carbohydrates throughout the day to avoid sharp spikes and drops in blood sugar levels.

- Incorporation of Proteins and Healthy Fats:

Protein and healthy fats are essential components of a balanced diet for people with diabetes. Protein helps maintain satiety and muscle mass, while healthy fats, such as those found in avocados, nuts, and olive oil, are beneficial for heart health. By choosing lean sources of protein and healthy fats, you can maintain a proper balance in your diet.

- Fiber and Micronutrients:

Dietary fiber is essential for digestion and can help control blood glucose levels. Fiber-rich foods, such as fruits, vegetables, legumes, and whole grains, should be an integral part of your daily diet. Additionally, it is crucial to ensure you get enough vitamins and minerals through a variety of foods to maintain overall health and well-being.

- Portion Sizes and Calorie Control:

Portion sizes and calorie control are important aspects of meal planning for people with diabetes. Controlling portion sizes helps avoid excess calories and can aid in weight management, which in turn improves insulin sensitivity. It is important to learn to read food labels and understand recommended serving sizes to avoid consuming more calories than necessary.

- The Importance of Education and Support:

Education about meal planning and a balanced diet is essential for people with diabetes. Working with a registered dietitian or diabetes educator can provide personalized guidance on how to create a meal plan suitable for individual needs. Additionally, emotional support and understanding of the immediate environment are vital to maintaining motivation and commitment to a healthy diet.

Meal planning and a balanced diet are cornerstones in effective diabetes management. By choosing foods carefully, controlling carbohydrates, incorporating protein and healthy fats, and paying attention to portion sizes, people with diabetes can maintain stable blood glucose levels and improve their quality of life. With education, support and commitment, it is possible to enjoy a delicious, balanced diet while effectively managing diabetes.

4.2 Exercise and physical activity: Benefits

Exercise and physical activity play a vital role in managing diabetes. For people with this chronic condition, incorporating regular exercise into their daily routine not only improves physical health, but also has positive impacts on mental and emotional health. Here, we will explore the significant benefits of exercise and physical activity for people with diabetes.

- Control of Blood Glucose Levels:

One of the most important benefits of exercise for people with diabetes is its ability to control blood glucose levels. During physical activity, muscles use glucose as an energy source, which lowers blood sugar levels. Additionally, exercise improves insulin sensitivity, allowing the body's cells to absorb glucose more efficiently. The combination of these effects can help keep glucose levels in a healthy range.

- Improved Insulin Sensitivity:

Insulin sensitivity is crucial for people with diabetes, especially those with type 2 diabetes, where the body's cells do not respond properly to insulin. Regular exercise improves insulin sensitivity, meaning cells can use insulin more effectively to absorb glucose. This helps reduce insulin resistance and contributes to long-term control of diabetes.

- Weight Management and Stress Reduction:

Exercise is a powerful tool for weight management. Maintaining a healthy weight is crucial for people with diabetes, as excess weight can worsen insulin resistance. Additionally, regular exercise helps reduce stress, a factor that can negatively affect blood glucose levels. The constant practice of physical activities can significantly contribute to reducing stress, thus improving general well-being.

- Improved Cardiovascular Health:

People with diabetes have a higher risk of heart disease. Regular exercise strengthens the heart, improves blood circulation and reduces blood pressure, which contributes to cardiovascular health. By maintaining a healthy heart, you reduce your chances of developing heart complications associated with diabetes.

- Increased Energy and Improved Sleep:

Regular exercise increases energy levels and improves sleep quality. People with diabetes often experience fatigue due to imbalances in blood glucose levels. Regular physical activity helps combat fatigue and improves sleep, leading to higher energy levels and an overall sense of well-being.

- Encouragement for an Active Lifestyle:

In addition to the physical benefits, exercise can inspire an overall active lifestyle. Engaging in regular physical activity can motivate people to seek out other forms of exercise, such as walking, swimming, or playing sports. This encourages a long-term healthy and active lifestyle.

Exercise and physical activity offer a variety of benefits for people with diabetes. From controlling blood glucose levels and improving insulin sensitivity to managing weight and improving cardiovascular health, regular exercise is a powerful tool in the effective management of diabetes. In addition, it contributes to emotional well-being and increased energy, promoting an active and healthy lifestyle for those living with this chronic condition.

4.3 Stress management and sleep

Stress management and sleep are vital aspects of diabetes care. For people living with this chronic condition, stress can negatively affect blood glucose levels, while lack of adequate sleep can influence insulin resistance and appetite control. Learning to manage stress and improving sleep quality are essential steps to maintaining balance in life and ensuring effective diabetes management.

- Stress and Blood Glucose:

Stress can trigger the release of stress hormones, such as cortisol and adrenaline, which raise blood glucose levels. In people with diabetes, this increase can make it difficult to control blood sugar levels. Additionally, stress often leads to unhealthy habits, such as emotional eating or lack of exercise, which can make the situation worse. Therefore, it is essential to adopt strategies to reduce stress and promote relaxation.

- Stress Management Techniques:

There are numerous stress management techniques that people with diabetes can incorporate into their daily lives. Meditation, deep breathing, yoga and tai Chi are effective practices that help reduce the body's response to stress. These techniques not only decrease cortisol and adrenaline levels, but also improve the overall feeling of well-being. Additionally, regularly engaging in recreational activities, such as reading, gardening, or music, can provide an escape from daily stress and improve mood.

- Sleep and Insulin Resistance:

Lack of adequate sleep can affect the way the body uses insulin, leading to increased resistance to this hormone. Insulin resistance makes it difficult for the body's cells to absorb glucose efficiently, which can increase blood sugar levels. Additionally, sleep deprivation can increase cravings for foods high in carbohydrates and sugars, further complicating blood sugar control.

- Improved Sleep Quality:

Improving sleep quality is essential for people with diabetes. Establishing a regular sleep routine, creating a sleep-friendly environment, and avoiding electronic stimulation before bed are practices that can improve sleep quality. Additionally, maintaining a cool, dark temperature in the bedroom, as well as investing in a comfortable mattress and pillows, can contribute significantly to restful sleep.

- Emotional Impact of Stress and Lack of Sleep:

Stress and lack of sleep can also affect mood and emotional health. People with diabetes may experience anxiety or depression related to managing their condition. Therefore, it is important to address both stress and lack of sleep to maintain mental and emotional health. Seeking support in the form of cognitive behavioral therapy, support groups, or speaking with a mental health professional can be beneficial in managing the emotional impact of stress and insufficient sleep.

Stress management and adequate sleep are crucial components of diabetes care. Adopting stress management techniques, improving sleep quality, and addressing the emotional impact of stress and lack of sleep are essential steps to maintaining balance in life and ensuring effective diabetes management. By incorporating these practices into daily routines, people with diabetes can improve their quality of life and promote more effective management of their chronic condition.

CHAPTER 5: Treatments and Medications

5.1 Medications to Control Blood Sugar

For many people with diabetes, effective blood sugar control is essential to living a healthy, active life. In addition to diet, exercise, and other lifestyle changes, medications play a crucial role in diabetes management. There are several types of medications designed to help control blood glucose levels, each with its unique mechanism of action and specific benefits.

- Oral Medications:

Oral medications are commonly prescribed for people with type 2 diabetes. These medications help lower blood glucose levels in several ways. Some stimulate the pancreas to release more insulin, while others improve insulin sensitivity or reduce the amount of glucose released by the liver. Oral medications are convenient and easy to take, making them a popular choice for many patients.

- Insulin:

Insulin is essential for people with type 1 diabetes and, in some cases, for people with advanced type 2 diabetes. Insulin is a hormone that allows the body's cells to absorb glucose from the blood to use for energy. There are several types of insulin available, varying in their speed of action and duration. Some are given before meals to help control the rise in glucose after eating, while others are used to maintain stable blood sugar levels throughout the day.

- Insulin Injectable Medications :

In addition to insulin, there are injectable medications that are not insulin-based but that help control blood glucose levels. These medications are often used in combination with other treatments to improve blood sugar control. Some of them work by reducing the amount of glucose released by the liver, while others help the kidneys eliminate excess glucose through urine.

- Incretin Medications :

Incretins are natural hormones in the body that help regulate blood glucose levels. Incretin medications , such as GLP-1 receptor agonists and DPP-4 inhibitors, mimic the effect of natural incretins . These medications stimulate the release of insulin and reduce the amount of glucose released by the liver after meals. Additionally, they may help reduce appetite and promote weight loss in some patients.

- SGLT-2 Medications:

cotransporter 2 (SGLT-2) inhibitors are a class of medications that help the kidneys get rid of excess glucose through urine. This helps reduce blood sugar levels. Additionally, these medications may have cardiovascular and kidney benefits in patients with diabetes and heart or kidney disease.

Medications to control blood sugar are essential tools in managing diabetes. Each patient is unique, so it is crucial to work closely with a healthcare professional to determine the appropriate treatment. With the right combination of medications, diet, exercise, and regular monitoring, people with diabetes can lead active, healthy lives, keeping blood glucose levels within a target range and reducing the risk of long-term complications. It is essential to follow the instructions of the medical team and make adjustments to the treatment plan as necessary to ensure optimal diabetes control and a better quality of life.

5.2 Insulin and its administration

Insulin is a vital hormone for the human body. It is produced in the pancreas and plays a fundamental role in glucose metabolism, allowing cells to absorb and use sugar as an energy source. For people with type 1 diabetes and some people with type 2 diabetes, external insulin becomes a daily necessity to maintain blood glucose levels within a healthy range. Understanding insulin, its delivery, and its impact on the body is essential for effective diabetes management.

- Types of Insulin:

There are several types of insulin, differentiated by their speed of action and duration. Rapid-acting insulin starts working almost immediately and has a short duration, making it ideal for controlling sugar levels after meals. Intermediate-acting insulin has a slower onset and longer duration, being useful for maintaining stable glucose levels between meals and overnight. Additionally, there are long-acting insulins that provide continuous coverage throughout the day.

- Forms of Administration:

Insulin administration can be done through injections or through continuous infusion devices, such as insulin pumps. Injections are given into specific areas of the body, such as the abdomen, thighs, or buttocks, using syringes, insulin pens, or automatic injection devices. Insulin pumps, on the other hand, are small electronic devices that continuously deliver insulin through a subcutaneous catheter. These devices offer flexibility in dosing and pattern administration, allowing for more precise control of blood glucose levels.

- Factors to Consider in Administration:

Several factors must be taken into account when administering insulin. These include the amount of carbohydrates in meals, physical activity, stress, illnesses, and other medications the person may be taking. The insulin dose must be adjusted based on these factors to maintain stable blood sugar levels. Additionally, rotating injection sites is crucial to prevent the buildup of scar tissue in specific areas of the body, which could affect insulin absorption.

- Education and Support:

It is essential to receive proper education on insulin administration and how to adjust doses based on individual needs. Health care professionals, such as diabetes educators or nurse practitioners, can provide detailed guidance on administration techniques, site rotation, and handling special situations, such as illness or strenuous exercise. Additionally, having a support system, whether in the form of family, friends, or online support groups, can help people with diabetes cope with the emotional and practical challenges associated with taking insulin.

Insulin and its effective administration are essential for people with diabetes who require this hormone to control their blood sugar levels. Understanding the different types of insulin, the forms of administration and the factors that affect doses are essential knowledge for adequate management of the disease. Education, support and open communication with the healthcare team are key to ensuring that people with diabetes use insulin safely and effectively, allowing them to lead full and active lives while optimally managing their condition. With the right knowledge and the right support, people with diabetes can live healthy, productive lives while managing their disease effectively and safely.

5.3 Complementary Therapies

In the management of diabetes, complementary therapies offer a holistic approach that goes beyond conventional medical treatments. These therapies focus on physical, mental and emotional well-being, and can play an important role in controlling blood glucose levels, managing stress and improving quality of life. Although it is essential to consult a health professional before incorporating any complementary therapies, many people with diabetes have found significant benefits from integrating these practices into their daily routine.

- Acupuncture:

Acupuncture is an ancient therapy originating from traditional Chinese medicine that involves inserting thin needles into specific points on the body. It is believed that acupuncture can help balance the body's energy, which can improve insulin sensitivity and reduce stress levels. Some people with diabetes have experienced a decrease in blood glucose levels and an improvement in sleep quality after receiving regular acupuncture treatments.

- Yoga and Tai Chi:

Yoga and tai Chi are physical and mental practices that combine movement, breathing and meditation. These disciplines have been shown to reduce stress levels and improve flexibility and balance. For people with diabetes, regular yoga or tai practice Chi can help maintain a healthy weight, improve circulation, and promote an overall sense of well-being. Additionally, these activities can be adapted for people of all ages and fitness levels.

- Meditation and Mindfulness :

Meditation and mindfulness are practices that focus on concentration and awareness of the present moment. These techniques have been shown to reduce stress levels and improve emotional control. For people with diabetes, chronic stress can negatively affect blood glucose levels, so learning to manage stress through meditation and mindfulness can be beneficial . Meditation can also help improve sleep quality, which is crucial for maintaining stable blood sugar levels.

- Nutritional supplements:

Some nutritional supplements, such as omega-3, chromium, and magnesium, have been studied for their possible benefits in diabetes management. Omega-3, found in fish oils, may have anti-inflammatory effects and improve insulin sensitivity. Chromium and magnesium have also been shown to influence blood glucose levels. However, it is important to speak with a health professional before starting any supplement to make sure it is safe and suitable for your situation.

- Massage Therapy:

Therapeutic massages not only provide relaxation, but can also improve blood circulation and reduce stress. For people with diabetes, a regular massage can help relieve muscle tension and promote relaxation, which can contribute to overall well-being. Additionally, massages can improve sleep quality and help relieve pain and discomfort associated with diabetic neuropathy.

Complementary therapies offer valuable options for people with diabetes seeking a comprehensive approach to managing their condition. It is always important to speak with a health professional before starting any complementary therapy to make sure it is safe and appropriate for your specific situation. By integrating these practices into their daily routine, people with diabetes can experience significant benefits in terms of blood glucose control, stress reduction and improved quality of life, thus contributing to more effective and satisfactory management of their condition.

CHAPTER 6: Prevention

6.1 Prevention and Control of Complications

Diabetes is a chronic disease that, if not properly controlled, can lead to a number of serious complications. However, with careful management and a comprehensive approach to self-care, many of these complications can be prevented or effectively managed. It is essential for people with diabetes to understand the risks and take preventive measures to ensure a long and healthy life.

- Control of Blood Glucose Levels:

Maintaining blood glucose levels within a target range is critical to preventing diabetes-related complications. Regular monitoring of blood sugar levels, along with appropriate administration of insulin and/or oral medications, helps prevent sharp spikes and drops in blood glucose, thereby reducing the risk of long-term complications.

- Control of blood pressure:

People with diabetes have a higher risk of developing high blood pressure. High blood pressure can damage blood vessels and increase the risk of heart disease, stroke, and kidney disease. It is essential to control blood pressure through lifestyle changes and, if necessary, medications prescribed by a health professional.

- Maintaining Healthy Body Weight:

Overweight and obesity are significant risk factors for diabetes complications. Maintaining a healthy body weight through a balanced diet and regular exercise helps improve insulin sensitivity and prevent heart disease, hypertension, and joint problems, among other complications associated with excess weight.

- Control of Cholesterol and Triglycerides:

People with diabetes are at increased risk of developing high blood cholesterol and triglycerides, which can increase the risk of heart disease. Controlling LDL cholesterol ("bad cholesterol") levels and increasing HDL cholesterol ("good cholesterol") levels through diet and, if necessary, medications, is essential for reducing the risk of heart disease and other complications. .

- Foot Care:

Peripheral neuropathy and poor blood circulation, common in people with diabetes, can increase the risk of foot ulcers and infections. It is crucial to inspect your feet regularly, keep the skin clean and well hydrated, wear appropriate footwear, and consult a podiatrist to avoid foot complications.

- Regular Medical Exams:

Carrying out regular medical examinations is essential to detect and control early complications. Eye exams can help prevent vision problems, while regular blood and urine tests can provide crucial information about kidney function and other health indicators.

- Healthy life style:

Adopting a healthy lifestyle that includes a balanced diet, regular exercise, abstinence from tobacco and moderate alcohol consumption can make a big difference in preventing and managing diabetes complications. These healthy habits not only help keep blood glucose levels under control, but also promote cardiovascular and emotional health.

Prevention and control of complications in diabetes require a comprehensive approach that includes careful management of blood glucose levels, attention to blood pressure, control of cholesterol and triglycerides, foot care, examinations regular doctors and adopting a healthy lifestyle. By taking proactive measures and working closely with a healthcare team, people with diabetes can significantly reduce the risk of complications and enjoy a full, active life, keeping the disease under control and maximizing their overall well-being.

6.2 Blood pressure and cholesterol monitoring

Regular monitoring of blood pressure and cholesterol levels is essential for people with diabetes, as both factors are closely related to the risk of heart and vascular complications. Diabetes can negatively affect the cardiovascular system, increasing the likelihood of developing high blood pressure and high cholesterol levels, which in turn can increase the risk of heart disease and stroke. That is why it is essential to understand the importance of constant monitoring and how these measures contribute to the effective management of diabetes.

- Blood pressure:

Hypertension, or high blood pressure, is a common complication in people with diabetes. High blood pressure can damage blood vessels and increase the risk of heart disease, stroke, and kidney disease. For this reason, it is recommended that people with diabetes monitor their blood pressure regularly, at home and in clinical settings. Target blood pressure values for people with diabetes are generally below 130/80 mm Hg. Regular monitoring makes it possible to detect changes in blood pressure and take preventive measures or adjust treatment if necessary.

- Cholesterol Levels:

Cholesterol is a fatty substance found in the blood and is essential for building cells and hormones in the body. However, high levels of certain types of cholesterol, such as LDL ("bad cholesterol"), can increase the risk of plaque buildup in the arteries, which hinders blood flow and increases the risk of heart disease. People with diabetes should pay special attention to their cholesterol levels and work to keep them within a healthy range. Optimal levels vary depending on the individual clinical situation, so it is important to discuss specific goals with a healthcare professional.

- How to Monitor Blood Pressure and Cholesterol:

Blood pressure monitoring can be done at home with a digital blood pressure monitor. It is advisable to take blood pressure in a quiet environment and follow the device manufacturer's instructions. Additionally, people with diabetes should undergo regular blood pressure screenings in doctors' offices for accurate measurements and long-term monitoring.

To measure cholesterol levels, blood tests, known as lipid profiles, are performed. These tests measure levels of total cholesterol, LDL cholesterol, HDL cholesterol ("good cholesterol"), and triglycerides. The results of these tests provide crucial information about cardiovascular risk and help guide treatment and lifestyle modifications.

- Interventions to Control Blood Pressure and Cholesterol:

If elevated blood pressure or cholesterol levels are detected, there are various interventions that can help control these risk factors. Changes in diet, increased physical activity, and, in some cases, medications prescribed by a healthcare professional are common measures. Adopting a low-sodium diet rich in fruits, vegetables, whole grains, and healthy fats can help control both blood pressure and cholesterol levels.

In conclusion, regular monitoring of blood pressure and cholesterol levels is essential for the effective management of diabetes and the prevention of complications related to the heart and blood vessels. By staying alert to these risk factors and working closely with a healthcare team, people with diabetes can take proactive steps to protect their cardiovascular health and improve their quality of life. Continued surveillance and appropriate interventions are critical steps toward a healthier, more active future for those living with diabetes.

6.3 Eye problems and their prevention

Eye problems are a common complication in people with diabetes, and prevention plays a crucial role in maintaining long-term vision health. Diabetes can affect the eyes in a variety of ways, from vision disturbances to more serious eye diseases that can lead to vision loss. It is essential to understand the risks, take preventive measures, and perform regular eye exams to protect your vision and preserve quality of life.

Vision Risks in People with Diabetes:

- **Diabetic Retinopathy:** This is a specific ocular complication of diabetes. Diabetic retinopathy develops when high blood glucose levels damage the blood vessels in the retina, the part of the eye that captures light. This can lead to vision loss if not properly controlled.
- **Cataracts:** People with diabetes are at increased risk of developing cataracts, a clouding of the eye's lens that can cause blurred vision and eventual vision loss.
- **Glaucoma:** People with diabetes also have an increased risk of glaucoma, an eye disease that damages the optic nerve and can lead to loss of peripheral vision.
- **Dry Eye:** Diabetes can cause dry eye, a condition in which the eyes do not produce enough tears to keep the surface of the eye lubricated, which can cause discomfort and blurred vision.

Precautionary measures:

- **Blood Glucose Control:** Maintaining blood glucose levels within a target range is essential to prevent eye problems. Stability in blood sugar levels helps reduce the risk of diabetic retinopathy and other eye complications.

- **Regular Eye Exams:** People with diabetes should have regular eye exams at least once a year, even if they do not experience visual symptoms. These exams allow eye problems to be detected in early stages, when they are most treatable.
- **Blood Pressure and Cholesterol Under Control:** Maintaining healthy blood pressure and cholesterol levels is also important to prevent diabetes-related eye diseases. High blood pressure and high cholesterol levels can negatively affect eye health.
- **Sun Protection:** Prolonged exposure to UV rays can increase the risk of cataracts. Wearing sunglasses with UV protection helps protect your eyes from ultraviolet radiation.
- **Avoid Tobacco:** Smoking increases the risk of developing eye problems, including diabetic retinopathy. Quitting smoking can significantly reduce this risk.
- **Stress Management:** Chronic stress can affect eye health. Practicing stress management techniques, such as meditation and relaxation, can help reduce this risk.

Prevention and eye care are essential for people with diabetes. By keeping blood glucose levels under control, undergoing regular eye exams and adopting a healthy lifestyle, the risks of diabetes-related eye problems can be significantly reduced. Sight is an invaluable sense, and taking care of your eyes is essential to enjoying a clear life without visual complications. By taking preventative measures and working collaboratively with a healthcare team, people with diabetes can preserve their vision and improve their quality of life, allowing them to face the future with confidence and visual clarity.

CHAPTER 7: Emotional and psychological support

―――――

7.1 Tips for Family and Friends Support

Support from family and friends is invaluable for people living with diabetes. The understanding, care and patience of loved ones play a crucial role in the effective management of this chronic condition. When friends and family provide strong support, people with diabetes can face everyday challenges with greater confidence and optimism. Here are some tips to help create a positive and supportive environment:

Education and Awareness:

- Invite your friends and family to learn about diabetes. The more they understand the condition, the better they will be able to support you.
- Share trusted resources, books, and educational websites so they can educate themselves about the medical and emotional aspects of diabetes.

Promote a Healthy Lifestyle:

- Encourage your loved ones to adopt a healthy lifestyle with you. Exercising together and preparing balanced meals can be a shared and beneficial experience for everyone.
- Organize family activities that involve physical activity, such as walks or bike rides, to encourage an active lifestyle for everyone.

Emotional Support:

- Diabetes can be emotionally challenging. Thank your loved ones for being there for you emotionally and express your feelings and needs to them.

- Consider joining online or in-person support groups, where you and your loved ones can share experiences and get guidance.

Open Communication:

- Encourage open and honest communication. Let them know how you feel and what you need, either emotionally or practically, to manage your diabetes.
- Listen to their concerns too. Sometimes loved ones may feel helpless and may need space to share their emotions and questions.

Respect and Empathy:

- Build empathy and respect for your diabetes-related challenges and achievements. Celebrate small wins together and recognize continued efforts.
- Remember that support also means respecting your decisions and treatments. Each person with diabetes has a unique approach to managing their condition.

Participation in Care:

- Invite your loved ones to participate in your daily care if they are willing. They can learn how to administer insulin, help you monitor your glucose levels, or simply be present during doctor's appointments.
- Make sure they feel valued and appreciated for their contribution to managing your diabetes.

Celebrate Accomplishments Together:

- Celebrate achievements together, whether big or small. It could be reaching a blood glucose goal, maintaining a healthy lifestyle for a specific period, or simply facing a challenging day successfully.
- These celebrations reinforce mutual support and create a sense of community and shared achievement.

Ultimately, family and friend support not only improves diabetes management, but also strengthens emotional bonds. Diabetes can be challenging, but with the right love, understanding and support, people living with this condition can face it with determination and quality of life. By building a strong supportive environment, people with diabetes and their loved ones can face challenges together, celebrate achievements, and navigate this journey in a positive and hopeful way.

7.2 Dealing with Depression and Anxiety

Diabetes not only affects the physical body, but also the mental and emotional well-being of people living with this chronic condition. Depression and anxiety are common challenges that can arise due to the daily demands of diabetes management. It is essential to address these issues holistically to ensure a comprehensive approach to well-being.

Recognize Feelings:

- It is important to recognize and validate the feelings of sadness, frustration, and anxiety that can arise when facing diabetes. These feelings are natural and should not be ignored.

Seek Professional Support:

- Consider talking to a mental health professional, such as a psychologist or psychiatrist, who has experience treating people with diabetes. Cognitive behavioral therapy and supportive therapy may be beneficial in addressing emotional challenges.

Open Communication:

- Talk openly and honestly with your loved ones about your feelings. Open communication can ease emotional weight and foster a supportive environment.
- Encourage your loved ones to learn about diabetes and its emotional aspects so they can better understand your challenges.

Establish Healthy Routines:

- Establish regular sleep, exercise, and eating routines. A healthy lifestyle can help reduce anxiety and improve mood.
- Practice relaxation techniques, such as meditation and deep breathing, to reduce stress and anxiety.

Avoid Isolation:

- Avoid social isolation. Engage in activities and hobbies that you enjoy and that connect you with other people. Social support can have a positive impact on mood.

Set Realistic Goals:

- Set realistic goals for yourself in terms of diabetes management. Celebrating small achievements can improve self-esteem and reduce feelings of overwhelm .

Continuing Education:

- Learn as much as you can about diabetes and how to manage it effectively. The more you understand the condition, the better equipped you will be to deal with the emotional challenges that arise.

Avoid Guilt and Self-Judgement :

- Diabetes is not your fault. Avoid blaming yourself for the challenges you face. Self -acceptance and self-love are essential for emotional well-being.

Foster a Supportive Environment:

- Share your emotional needs with your loved ones and foster a supportive environment at home. The understanding and encouragement of your loved ones can make a big difference in your emotional well-being.

Practice Self-Care:

- Make time for yourself for activities that bring you joy and relaxation. Whether reading, listening to music, practicing hobbies or simply resting, self-care is essential for emotional well-being.

Dealing with depression and anxiety in the context of diabetes requires a compassionate and multidimensional approach. Seeking professional support, communicating openly and honestly, establishing healthy routines, and fostering a supportive environment are critical steps in addressing emotional challenges. With the right support and appropriate strategies, people with diabetes can address depression and anxiety, live full lives, and maintain emotional balance that contributes to their overall well-being.

7.3 Support Groups and Online Resources

When living with diabetes, having the right support is essential to face daily challenges and maintain a positive mindset. Support groups and online resources are valuable tools that can provide not only helpful information, but also a sense of community and emotional connection with people who share similar experiences. These groups and resources can make a big difference in managing diabetes, providing emotional support, practical guidance, and a space to share concerns and triumphs.

Online Community:

- Online platforms, such as discussion forums and social networks, offer spaces where people with diabetes can connect, share experiences and get emotional support. These environments allow you to ask questions, receive advice, and feel understood by others facing similar challenges.

Applications for Diabetes:

- There are numerous mobile applications designed specifically to help with diabetes management. These apps allow you to track glucose levels, diet, exercise and medication, offering instant feedback and reminders to maintain constant control.

Diabetes Association Websites:

- Diabetes associations, both locally and internationally, often have websites with educational resources, informative articles, and links to online support groups. These websites offer reliable, up-to-date information on all aspects of diabetes, from nutrition to the latest medical research.

Local Support Groups:

- Participating in local support groups provides the opportunity to interact face-to-face with people who live in the same community. These groups often host regular meetings where diabetes-related topics are discussed, practical advice is shared, and camaraderie is fostered.

Webinars and Podcasts :

- Online diabetes webinars and podcasts offer a convenient way to access valuable information . Diabetes experts and medical professionals often present webinars on a variety of topics, from glucose management technology to strategies to improve quality of life.

YouTube Channels:

- Many people and health professionals have created YouTube channels dedicated to diabetes. These channels offer educational videos, personal testimonials, and practical advice for living well with the condition. Watching videos can be an accessible and visual way to learn about diabetes.

Social networks:

- Social media offers a platform to follow influencers and diabetes experts. These profiles often share inspiring content, healthy recipes, exercise tips and motivational messages, creating a positive virtual community for those living with the disease.

Specific Groups for Types of Diabetes:

- There are specific support groups for different types of diabetes, such as type 1, type 2, and gestational diabetes. These groups allow people to interact with others who face similar challenges in terms of treatment and management of the disease.

Participating in support groups and using online resources not only provides practical knowledge about diabetes management, but also provides a sense of community and belonging. By connecting with others who understand the struggles and triumphs associated with diabetes, people can find encouragement, inspiration, and motivation to stay on the path of self-care. These groups and resources are a reminder that you are not alone in your journey and that there is a vast world of support waiting for you online and in your local communities.

CHAPTER 8: Living Fully with Diabetes

8.1 Travel and Socialize with Diabetes

Travel and socializing are activities that enrich our lives, but when living with diabetes, they can present unique challenges. However, with proper planning and a conscious approach, it is possible to fully enjoy these experiences while maintaining control over the condition. Here are tips for traveling and socializing with diabetes safely and without complications:

Advance Planning:

- Before traveling or attending social events, make sure you have a sufficient supply of medications, test strips, insulin, and other supplies needed for your trip or outing. Always carry more supplies with you than you think you will need in an emergency.
- Consult your doctor before traveling to adjust any medications or insulin regimens based on time zone differences and planned activities.

Medic Alert and Documentation:

- Wear a medical identification bracelet or carry a medical information card stating that you have diabetes and emergency contact details. In an emergency, this information can be vital for health professionals.

Meal Planning:

- Research places to eat at your destination and look for healthy and balanced options. If you are attending a social gathering or event, consider talking to the organizers about your dietary needs. Many places can prepare special meals if you notify them in advance.

Glucose Control and Monitoring:

- Keep track of your blood glucose levels and adjust your treatment as necessary. Always carry a glucose meter with you and monitor your levels regularly to avoid complications.

Exercise During the Trip:

- If you're going to be sitting for a long time during a trip, be sure to move regularly to maintain circulation and avoid blood sugar spikes. Get up, stretch your legs, and do some light exercises to avoid prolonged inactivity.

Communication with Travel Companions or Friends:

- If you are traveling with friends or family, make sure they are aware of your condition and know how to help you in an emergency. Discuss warning signs of hypoglycemia or hyperglycemia so they can recognize potential symptoms.

Empathy and Understanding:

- When socializing, don't hesitate to explain your condition to friends and colleagues if necessary. Most people will be understanding and willing to help you if you need it.

Emergency Preparedness:

- Carry an emergency kit that includes glucagon, gel sugar, or glucose tablets in case of severe hypoglycemia. Also make sure you have an action plan in case of emergency and that your companions know the procedure to follow.

Adaptability and Patience:

- Situations can change quickly during a trip or social event. Maintain an adaptable and patient attitude to deal with any eventuality. Patience is key to facing unexpected challenges.

Enjoy the moment:

- Despite necessary precautions, don't let diabetes stop you from fully enjoying your travel and social experiences. With proper planning and proper care, you can live life without unnecessary limitations.

In short, traveling and socializing with diabetes requires a proactive and careful approach, but it doesn't have to be restrictive. With good planning, open communication, and proper condition management, you can enjoy every moment without unnecessary worries. Remember that you control diabetes, not the other way around. With a positive mindset and the right precautions, you can explore the world and enjoy social interactions in a safe and meaningful way.

8.2 Advice for Employment and Education

Diabetes should not be an obstacle to achieving your professional and educational goals. With proper management and a proactive approach, it is possible to excel in both the work and academic fields. Here are some tips to help you thrive in your career and education while living with diabetes:

Open Communication:

- Talk to your employer, teachers or classmates about your condition. Open communication is key so that people around you understand your needs and provide you with appropriate support at work or in the educational environment.

Planification and organization:

- Plan your days in advance. Establish regular times for meals and blood glucose measurements. Organize your tasks and responsibilities to avoid stressful last-minute situations.

Carry an Emergency Kit:

- At work or school, always carry an emergency kit containing glucagon, sugar gel, and any other medications or equipment needed in case of a hypoglycemic crisis .

Know your Rights:

- Research and understand your employment or educational rights related to diabetes. In many countries, there are laws that protect people with medical conditions by ensuring reasonable accommodations in the work or educational environment.

Continuing Education:

- Educate your co-workers or classmates about diabetes. The more they understand, the better they will be able to help you in emergency situations and the more understanding they will be of your needs.

Reasonable Accommodations:

- Request reasonable accommodations if you need them. This could include meal breaks, time off from classes or meetings to monitor your glucose, or even the option to work or study from home if possible.

Stress Management:

- Learn stress management techniques, such as meditation or deep breathing. Stress can affect blood glucose levels, so it is essential to maintain emotional balance.

Build a Support Network:

- Create a support network at work or school. Having colleagues or colleagues who understand your condition and are willing to help you if needed can provide great emotional relief.

Discreet Handling:

- Learn to manage your diabetes discreetly. Many devices and apps allow discreet blood glucose management , allowing you to monitor your levels without disrupting your daily routine too much.

Promotes Autonomy:

- As you become more competent in managing your diabetes, encourage autonomy. With practice and experience, you will learn to adjust your meals, medications, and activities based on your individual needs.

Remember, diabetes does not define your limits. With the right focus, continued education, and building a strong support network, you can achieve your goals in both work and education. Perseverance, knowledge, and self-care will empower you to meet challenges and thrive in your professional and academic aspirations.

8.3 Maintaining a Positive Attitude and Motivation

Diabetes can present significant challenges in daily life, but a positive and motivated attitude can make all the difference in how you deal with these challenges. An optimistic mindset not only improves your quality of life, but can also positively influence your physical and emotional health. Here are strategies to stay positive and motivated while facing diabetes:

Acceptance and Self-acceptance:

- Accepting your condition is the first step towards a positive mindset. Recognize that diabetes is just a part of who you are and does not define your worth as a person. Self -acceptance allows you to embrace your reality and work accordingly to live well with the illness.

Celebrate Small Accomplishments:

- Celebrate every achievement, no matter how small. Giving yourself an insulin shot correctly, maintaining stable blood glucose levels for a day, or following your diet plan are all achievements that deserve recognition. Celebrating these victories reinforces your motivation and self-esteem.

Positive Visualization:

- Practice positive visualization. Imagine your life with success and well-being, visualize yourself overcoming challenges and leading a full life. Positive visualization can increase your confidence and motivation to face the challenges of diabetes.

Set Realistic Goals:

- Set realistic and achievable goals for your diabetes management. These goals may be related to your glucose levels, your eating habits, or your exercise routine. Achieving small goals gives you a sense of accomplishment and boosts your motivation.

Practice Gratitude:

- Cultivate a sense of gratitude for the positive things in your life. Be grateful for the support of your loved ones, for medical advances, and for every day you feel well. Gratitude can shift your focus to what you have instead of what you lack.

Find Support and Community:

- Connect with other people living with diabetes. Joining support groups online or in person allows you to share experiences, receive helpful advice, and feel understood by people facing similar challenges.

Personal care:

- Spend time doing activities that bring you joy and relaxation. It can be anything from reading a book to pursuing a hobby or enjoying a walk in nature. Self-care nourishes your mind and spirit, strengthening your positive attitude.

Learn from Experiences:

- See challenges as learning opportunities. Every time you face an obstacle, ask yourself what you can learn from that experience. This approach helps you grow and find effective solutions to future challenges.

Surround yourself with Positivity:

- Surround yourself with positive people and environments. Avoid negativity and toxic influences in your life. Maintain relationships that support you and inspire you to stay positive.

Find Inspiration:

- Find inspiration from people who have overcome similar challenges. Read success stories, listen to motivational lectures, or follow people on social media who share positive and motivational messages. External inspiration can fuel your internal determination.

Maintaining a positive attitude and motivation in the fight against diabetes is essential to living a full and healthy life. An optimistic mindset not only helps you face challenges with resilience , but also improves your emotional and physical well-being. With the right attitude, the right support, and a positive approach to life, you can live with diabetes in a meaningful and fulfilling way. Mental strength and determination are your most powerful allies on this journey, helping you overcome obstacles and live each day with passion and positivity.

Conclusion

At this climax of our journey through "Manage Your Diabetes," I want to take a moment to express my gratitude and appreciation for having made it this far. They have traveled a path full of vital information, practical strategies and medical guidance, and for that, they deserve applause. Each page read represents a step towards empowerment, towards control and towards a healthier future. As you reach the end of this book, you have demonstrated an admirable dedication to educating yourself and facing diabetes head-on.

Throughout these pages, we have explored the intricate details of diabetes, from its diagnosis to daily management strategies. They have gained knowledge about the different types of diabetes, have understood the complexities of treatments and have learned to adapt their lifestyle to live fully, even with this chronic condition.

Let me be clear: facing diabetes is no easy task. It requires determination, patience, and a constant focus on self-care. They have shown impressive bravery in addressing the challenges of this disease with a positive and proactive mindset. They have learned to balance their blood glucose levels, navigated the complexities of diet and exercise, and faced each day with resilience and strength.

But this is not the end of your journey; It is simply a starting point for a continued life of self-empowerment and care. Every strategy they've learned, every medical advice they've internalized, and every lesson about emotional management of diabetes becomes valuable tools they'll carry with them into the future. The information you have absorbed here will give you the confidence and knowledge to face any challenge that arises.

I want you to know that you are not alone on this path. They have gained a deep understanding of their condition and have learned to be the strongest advocates for their own health. Every step you take forward should be filled with confidence and determination, knowing that you have the power to manage your diabetes and live a full life.

At this point, I want to express my sincere gratitude. Thank you for trusting this book as a source of guidance and support. Every word you have read has been carefully selected with the intention of providing you with the most accurate and useful information. I am deeply grateful for your dedication and commitment to your health, and I am inspired by your bravery in facing diabetes with determination and courage.

As you move forward in your lives after this book, I encourage you to continue to be proactive in your care. Continue to educate yourself, maintain open communication with your healthcare professionals, and above all, practice consistent self-care. You are the pillars of your own health and well-being, and your courage in facing diabetes will take you far.

In this closing, I want to wish you all the best on your continued journey. May each day be full of health, hope and determination. May they continue to live their lives with a positive mindset and a resilient attitude . I am confident that each of you has the power to bravely face diabetes and live an abundant and meaningful life.

With gratitude and admiration,

Dr. Paul Sterling

Don't miss out!

Visit the website below and you can sign up to receive emails whenever Dr Paul Sterling publishes a new book. There's no charge and no obligation.

https://books2read.com/r/B-A-OCJBB-ELPQC

BOOKS 2 READ

Connecting independent readers to independent writers.

Did you love *Managing Diabetes: Understanding and Controlling Type 1, Type 2, and Gestational Diabetes, Practical Strategies for Blood Sugar Management and Lifestyle Adaptation*? Then you should read *Mastering Gastritis: Comprehensive Guide to Understanding and Treating Acute, Chronic, and Erosive Gastritis, plus Stomach Inflammation Management*[1] by Dr Paul Sterling!

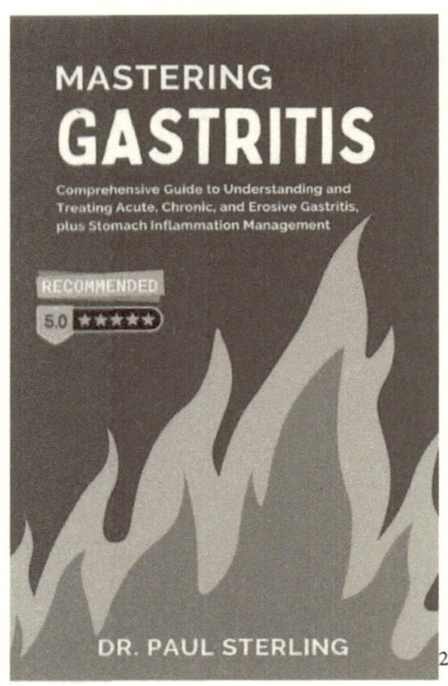

[2]

Unlock the secrets to optimal digestive health with "Mastering Gastric Wellness." This authoritative guide takes you on a journey through the complexities of gastric health, from understanding the nuances of gastritis to exploring advanced treatments and holistic approaches.

Why Choose "Mastering Gastric Wellness"?

In-Depth Knowledge: Dive deep into the world of gastric health, exploring various disorders, symptoms, and cutting-edge treatments, all explained in clear, concise language.Expert Guidance: Written by medical professionals, this book offers expert insights, evidence-based advice, and practical tips for managing gastric issues effectively.Holistic Solutions: Discover a range of solutions, from

---

1. https://books2read.com/u/38n7aZ

2. https://books2read.com/u/38n7aZ

pharmaceutical treatments to holistic approaches like yoga, acupuncture, and dietary interventions, ensuring you have a holistic toolkit for managing your digestive health.Empowerment and Support: Feel empowered to take control of your well-being. Learn how to recognize symptoms, make informed decisions, and foster mental and emotional resilience on your health journey.Time-Tested Wisdom: Benefit from centuries-old practices merged with the latest medical advancements, providing you with a well-rounded perspective on gastric health.Comprehensive and Accessible: Whether you're a medical professional, a patient, or someone interested in understanding digestive health, this book caters to all levels of knowledge, making complex medical information accessible to everyone.

Invest in Your Well-being Today!

"Mastering Gastric Wellness" is more than a book; it's your ultimate guide to digestive health. Equip yourself with the knowledge to lead a fulfilling life, free from the constraints of digestive issues. Purchase your copy now and embark on a transformative journey toward gastric wellness.

Note: Embrace the power of knowledge. Reviews and feedback are highly appreciated; your voice can inspire others on their journey to gastric wellness. Leave a review and be part of a supportive community committed to optimal health!

Also by Dr Paul Sterling

The Comprehensive Health Series
Mastering Gastritis: Comprehensive Guide to Understanding and Treating Acute, Chronic, and Erosive Gastritis, plus Stomach Inflammation Management
Managing Diabetes: Understanding and Controlling Type 1, Type 2, and Gestational Diabetes, Practical Strategies for Blood Sugar Management and Lifestyle Adaptation

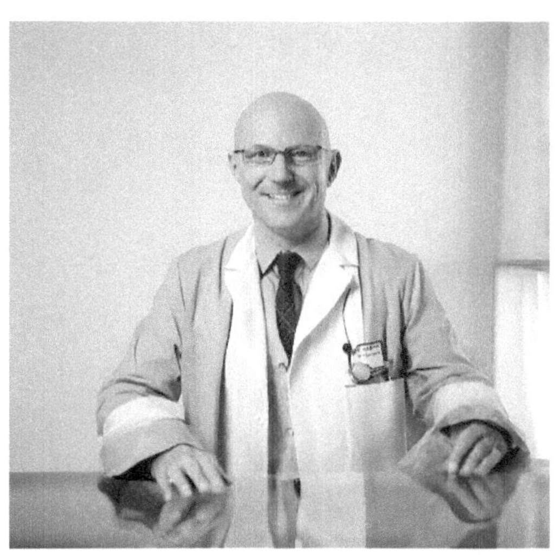

About the Author

Dr. Paul Sterling is a respected medical researcher and prolific author, standing as an influential leader in the field of medicine. With a multifaceted career spanning various specialties, he has made an indelible mark on medical innovation. His passionate dedication to research and profound knowledge in diverse areas of medicine has positioned him as a trailblazer in the medical field. Recognized with numerous awards and honors, Dr. Sterling is distinguished by his unwavering commitment to improving healthcare and patient well-being. Additionally, as an accomplished author, he has written numerous acclaimed books that educate and inspire people of all ages on health topics. His ability to communicate complex medical concepts in an accessible manner makes him an exemplary educator, whose legacy will endure thanks to his tireless pursuit of excellence in medicine and his dedication to enhancing the lives of others.

www.ingramcontent.com/pod-product-compliance
Lightning Source LLC
Chambersburg PA
CBHW030406160726
47992CB00007B/2985